STOPPING RESTLESS LEGS SYNDROME

BY CHET CUNNINGHAM

D1502408

 UNITED RESEARCH PUBLISHERS

Published by United Research Publishers

Copyright © 2000 by United Research Publishers

ISBN 1-887053-16-6

Printed and bound in the United States of America

The information in this publication is not intended to replace the advice of your physician. You should consult your doctor regarding any medical condition which concerns you. The material presented in this publication is intended to inform and educate the reader with a view to making some intelligent choices in pursuing the goal of living life in a healthy, vigorous manner.

Order additional copies from:
    United Research Publishers
    P. O. Box 232344
    Encinitas, CA 92023-2344

Or visit our website at:
    www.unitedresearchpubs.com

Full 90-day money back guarantee if not satisfied.

CONTENTS

WHAT IS RESTLESS LEGS
    SYNDROME? 5

WHAT IS PLMS? 9

WHAT CAUSES RLS? 11

DIAGNOSING RLS 15

TREATING RLS 21

MEDICAL TREATMENTS FOR RLS 31

COPING WITH RLS 41

JOIN AN RLS SUPPORT GROUP 49

THE RLS FOUNDATION 61

INDEX 63

WHAT IS RESTLESS LEGS SYNDROME?

Restless Legs Syndrome (RLS) is a serious physical problem that has for many years been ignored by some physicians, laughed at by others, and generally relegated to insignificant status. However, it is not a condition that is "all in your mind," or a result of some active imagination.

RLS is a definite neurological disorder that is finally being taken more seriously by the medical profession.

Generally RLS patients will fit these guidelines:

✔ **Mostly they will be women.**

✔ **Usually they will be fifty years or older.**

✔ **Almost always there will be bothersome—but not painful—sensations in the legs that result in an immediate need to move the limbs or to walk.**

✔ **These sensations in the legs—and sometimes the arms—almost always happen**

RLS is hard to describe since patients will often use different words.

5

when the patient is sitting or lying down.

4 The problem is worse in the evenings, when the patient may be sitting for long periods or lying down.

4 Sometimes there will be involuntary movement of the toes, feet or legs. This usually happens when the patient is in bed or after sitting for a long period of time.

4 Most RLS victims also have PLMS, or Periodic Limb Movement during Sleep. This limb movement is usually of the legs and can happen as often as every 25 seconds. Most people with PLMS are not aware of it, but it can cause a disturbed sleep that leaves the patient groggy and sleep deprived in the morning.

RLS can strike at anytime.

RLS is hard to describe since most patients use different words and have various feelings. Some say it's a gentle pain, others an ache, some say it's a creepy-crawly feeling, itching or even like pin pricks.

When a person with RLS has the creepy-crawly feeling in the legs, moving—such as walking or other exercise—usually will make the sensation lessen or even go away.

Patients sometimes report that they feel a minor annoyance like a feather brushing their legs. This might be for only a few seconds, or increase in intensity and length until the person desperately needs to get up and walk about or dance or do some leg exercises.

People with serious RLS say that the rapid onset of the feeling is scary. They say that the speed of the need to stamp their feet or get up and dance about or even run can at times become uncontrollable. One good thing here is that just as the sensations can come on quickly, they can also vanish rapidly.

6

If the patient isn't aware of the RLS problem, they often blame the symptoms on other things such as eating the wrong food, using shoes that don't fit, working too hard, or even not getting enough sleep.

No accurate count has been taken, but medical experts have estimated that some twelve million Americans suffer from RLS, and many of them don't even know what the letters mean, let alone what the affliction is that they have. They also don't know that there are medical and lifestyle ways to treat RLS and usually reduce the incidence—and sometimes even put it in remission.

RLS can strike at any time. Some get it when they sit at a desk at work. This can be disruptive to say the least. Others find it hits them when they sit down to watch a favorite TV show. Some women refuse to go to movies because they can't sit through a ninety minute show. The solution here is to rent a movie and use your video player at home.

Travel by car, plane or train also carries long periods of sitting down. We'll cover this later in the report.

The biggest problem with RLS right now is when physicians who should know better examine a patient and ridicule her and tell her that there is really nothing wrong. Some doctors tell the patient that he or she is a hypochondriac, or the problem is caused by stress, leg cramps, allergies, manic depression, muscle tautness, even "imaginary ills made up to get attention."

Doctors who do not understand RLS should get schooled in it immediately. If they don't, increasingly informed and vocal patients are going to give them in-office training that they may not like, but certainly need.

WHAT IS PLMS?

PLMS was briefly mentioned in the last section. It is Periodic Limb Movements in Sleep. It is often confused with RLS, but at the same time is closely associated with it. Some 80% of RLS patients also have PLMS. However many patients who have PLMS do not have RLS.

With PLMS the jerking legs may happen every twenty seconds or so during sleep. This might awaken the victim, and it might not. Often PLMS patients sleep through the movements and don't even know they have them. A bed partner who is constantly awakened by the movements, however, is acutely aware of the problem. In extreme cases this can lead to sleep deprivation for the spouse, and at the same time the affected person will be sleeping, but so groggy and un-rested in the morning that she wasn't sure how much sleep she had.

Many doctors think that PLMS may be a factor in up to 15% of those patients who complain of insomnia. The inability to get or stay asleep may be the PLMS of a partner, and they are not aware of it.

In some cases PLMS can happen when the patient is awake.

9

Daytime sleepiness in the PLMS patient or the spouse can often be tracked back to the PLMS. The sleep—even when continual—can be "disturbed" so that a deep sleep is not possible and the restorative powers of the body through deep sleep don't work. The victim will be sleepy during the day, and this can impair his or her driving or work performance.

In some cases the PLMS movements—in the legs or arms—can happen when the person is awake. When awake, the individual can walk or do some other activity to reduce or stop the PLMS movements.

Sleep experts say that there may be many people out there who have PLMS, but to a gentler degree so that he or she is not even aware of it. This would be especially true of a person sleeping alone where there's no one to learn of the leg kicking.

Is there any relation, genetically or otherwise between RLS and PLMS? The researchers are not sure. However the same medications can help to a certain degree in both situations. We'll cover this later.

WHAT CAUSES RLS ?

People who know say that just over one-third of all RLS cases are inherited. Males and females are equally affected by this inherited trait. The bad news is that the susceptibility for the condition is passed on to each succeeding generation. It's not like some inherited diseases that skip a generation every so often.

Only one parent needs to have RLS for the children of the union to get the disease. Which means if RLS runs in your family heritage and you don't get it, then your children will not get it if your spouse does not have the inherited trait.

One problem here is that RLS is usually active only in later years—50 to 60—and even then, it sometimes is so mild that the victims are never sure that they have the disease.

If the parent has the inherited form of RLS, it has been shown by research that half of the children

Children can get RLS.

11

Ferritin is a binding protein for essential iron

of that union will come down with RLS.

At the present time there is a push on to try to find the gene in the human system that is responsible for RLS. Blood is being evaluated from families with strong records of inherited RLS. Blood from people in other nations is also now being analyzed with the hope that the gene that causes the inherited RLS can be isolated and identified. Then there is a chance that some new therapies can be devised for the Restless Legs Syndrome and perhaps a cure found.

CHILDREN CAN GET RLS

We spoke of the onset of RLS as usually being in the fifties and sixties of adults. Until recently it was not thought that children ever had RLS. However, the kid's "growing pains" everyone talked about we now know may be a form of childhood RLS. The disease can show up in children in many ways: night jerks, leg pains, short attention span, hyperactivity, bedtime struggles, sleep walking, and even severe headaches.

A survey of adult RLS patients showed that 45% remembered symptoms of RLS that came about when they were children.

RLS is thought to be a factor in aggravating ADHD, or Attention Deficit Hyperactivity Disorder.

Researchers say that their work regarding childhood RLS is just starting. They need to do much more. But it could be a good signpost for parents who have children with "growing pains" to have a doctor who knows about RLS take a good long look at the child, and the child's activity and history. This is especially important if there is any record of hereditary RLS in the family.

SECONDARY CAUSES OF RLS

There may be secondary causes of RLS, which can aggravate the underlying RLS. Some of these triggers seem to create transient symptoms of RLS. For

12

example if you drink caffeine in any beverage such as coffee, tea, hot chocolate or most soft drinks, or even eat chocolate, you may have an increase in the symptoms of an underlying case of RLS. The good part here is that when you cut out this caffeine intake, the symptoms of RLS usually go away. However, even if it isn't the primary cause of your RLS, the caffeine will make the symptoms much worse.

PREGNANCY CAN DO IT

Another physical situation that can actually cause RLS is pregnancy. During the last few months of pregnancy, as many as 15% of mothers-to-be suffer from RLS. Your gynecologist should have told you about this, but if he or she didn't, pick it up now. In the later stages of pregnancy, the pressure on blood vessels leading to the legs can be such that it can bring on temporary RLS. There isn't a lot that can be done for the problem, except for the comfort methods of hot baths and some good walking exercise. The real relief comes with delivery, after which the symptoms of RLS usually vanish. Not always, but most of the time. A few will not lose their symptoms, and will need a doctor's care or medication.

On the same note, a woman's monthly cycle may result in a heavy blood loss, and a corresponding loss of iron. RLS seems to happen more frequently to women with a heavy blood flow during menstruation lasting five days or more. Hormonal changes here may also be a factor.

If your RLS symptoms worsen during this time, consult your doctor about checking your ferritin level. If it's below 50, he will give you iron pills or other help to bring it up to the minimum safe level of 50.

OTHER CAUSES OF RLS

For more than thirty years, doctors have known that anemia (low levels of iron in the blood) and

Several diseases adversely affect RLS.

13

vitamin deficiency have a bearing on RLS.

A low level of ferritin is reported in 25% of RLS and PLMS patients. Ferritin is a binding protein for iron. This level is one of the best gauges for how much iron your body has stored or has in its savings account. It is usually right for the ferritin level to be at least 50 for those with RLS. Iron influences how dopamine works in the brain. When it is low, it could contribute to disabling the dopamine system. If an RLS patient's level of ferritin is under 50, and work is done to raise it to 50 or above, there usually is a marked improvement in the RLS patient.

Warning: ferritin level is not included in most panels of blood work (such as a CBC) your doctor may order. It must be requested separately.

When an RLS or PLMS patient's ferritin level is below 50 an iron supplement usually is taken. A daily dose is one to three iron tablets of 65 mg of elemental iron and 325 mg of iron sulfate with Vitamin C added or taken separately. The Vitamin C helps the iron absorption.

Iron tablets can often cause constipation. If this happens, the RLS patient can consider taking Citrucel. One iron supplement, Niferex, is said to be less constipating.

Another idea here is to eat more foods that are high in iron. One brand of black strap molasses has 20% of the RDA for iron in one tablespoon. The dark meat of chicken has three times the iron as the white meat. Caffeine, high fiber foods and calcium supplements can reduce iron absorption.

There is a group of diseases that can aggravate or in some cases cause RLS. Nobody is sure just why. These other physical conditions—including diabetes, damage to nerves in the hands and feet (peripheral neuropathy), Parkinson's disease, neuropathy, alcoholism, rheumatoid arthritis and kidney disease—all can result in longer-lasting RLS. You're not going to cure these problems, but by working with your doctors to make them better, you could also help reduce the severity of your RLS.

Other diseases that find RLS showing up more frequently include amylodosis, Attention Deficit Hyperactivity Disorder, fibromyalgia, lumbosacral radiculopathy, spinal lesions, spine, back or head injury, lyme disease, stomach surgery, Tourette's syndrome, and multiple sclerosis. Here again, helping the other disease may help reduce or eliminate the RLS.

Many RLS patients report that they find their symptoms worse when they have a full bladder.

Idiopathic is a great descriptive word in medicine that should have a wider use. It simply means that there is no known cause for a disease or a physical problem. This is another way for the doctors to say that you have no physical ailment or deficiency that could have caused your RLS, and you have no history of hereditary RLS, therefore the cause is idiopathic.

DIAGNOSING RLS

Older patients today who have RLS can tell you horror stories about how they were misdiagnosed for many years. Until only a few years ago, there was little known or understood about RLS. Doctors had never heard of it.

Time after time, doctors would tell patients they had nothing wrong with them. All tests came back negative. They were making up the pains and problems, they were hypochondriacs, and they were playing games with the doctor's valuable time.

Until about ten years ago, few medical schools taught any courses about RLS, what it was or how to treat it. Even today most older doctors have little understanding of the problem, unless they have been alert or had a patient with RLS and bothered to research it.

Today diagnosing RLS is still not much easier. There is no laboratory test to do the job. No hard and fast method that can pronounce a yes or no diagnosis.

Diagnosis is done strictly by symptoms that the patient tells the doctor. Also by a search of the

Diagnosis of RLS is done strictly by symptoms.

patient's hereditary background to find any other family members who might have had RLS, and a check of the patient's physical condition to see if there are any underlying problems that might be contributing to the RLS.

The Restless Legs Syndrome Foundation has prepared a list for a person to go through to decide if he or she should contact a healthcare specialist to determine if there is RLS.

1. **Before I fall asleep, I develop an unpleasant or creepy, crawly sensation in my legs. Sometimes, I get this same feeling in other parts of my body.**

2. **In order to relieve this sensation, I get up and walk, do deep knee bends, take a hot or cold bath, massage my legs, or perform some other activity.**

3. **I develop this unpleasant or creepy, crawly sensation when I sit for a period of time such as when watching television or a movie, riding in the car, attending the theater or my place of worship, or participating in a meeting.**

4. **The sensations bother me most in the evening or at night.**

5. **No medical tests have revealed a cause for my sensations.**

6. **I have family members who experience these same sensations.**

7. **My bed partner tells me that I jerk my legs or my arms when I am asleep; sometimes I have involuntary leg jerks when I am awake.**

8. **I often have trouble falling asleep or staying asleep.**

9. I frequently feel tired or fatigued during the day.

If you answer yes to most of these questions, you definitely should consult your physician and tell her what is happening. Make her listen to you before she starts prescribing. Make her understand what is happening.

The best argument you have when talking to a doctor is simply to know more about RLS than he does. Your job first may be to educate the doctor about RLS, then show that there are three generations of women in your family who have had RLS and didn't know what it was, that you sometimes are low on iron and have been anemic in the past. Lay out all of the symptoms that you can, so he can understand what the basics of RLS entail. You need his cooperation so you can get the prescriptions that you need. Remember that RLS is treatable—it is not curable. With proper treatment and life style changes, you should be able to reduce the symptoms so you can get a good night's sleep.

TREATING RLS

To begin, be assured that RLS is an intermittent and chronic disease for which there is no outright cure, and for which there must be treatment over many years.

Since the 1980s there have been a number of double-blind studies done on various drugs in an attempt to find the right ones for RLS. Some of these were done in combination with tests on patients with PLMS, Periodic Limb Movements in Sleep, which we have talked about before: since both seem to have some of the same characteristics, perhaps the same drug would treat them both.

Today there are several drugs that can help RLS, and in the future more will be tested and put to use. The ultimate hope for RLS patients is to find the gene that causes the problem. This could open many new methods of treatment including the chance of a genetic cure so family members downstream would not have the potential for the disease.

Many physicians are aware that some patients

Chances are your doctor won't know anything about RLS.

do not need medications to keep their RLS in check. These patients can often make their symptoms manageable by doing the proper amount of exercise each day, avoiding caffeine, or having a quick five minutes on an exercise bike or a hot shower before bedtime. Others may look to a wide group of dietary, holistic or herbal practices that keep their RLS at a workable level where they can get a good eight hours of sleep a night.

Other patients may need a regimen of medications over a period of years to keep their symptoms in check so they can live a much more nearly normal life, and without serious side effects.

SOME GUIDELINES FOR TREATING RLS

The starting point for treating your RLS is to search out a doctor who knows about RLS, knows how to treat it, and with whom you can get along and trust. Not all physicians know about RLS or know how to treat it. It may take some shopping around, and talking to any friends who have RLS. One good spot to check on doctors is at a local RLS support group. Join the group and find out which doctors do the best job, then go and see them.

If you're in an HMO it will be tougher. You've been assigned a general practitioner. Chances are he won't know anything about RLS. If he doesn't, ask him who in the organization is best informed about RLS and who can help you. There should be at least one person in a large HMO who knows about RLS.

In many cases these days, a local doctor or even an HMO GP can obtain expert help on RLS from a real expert half a nation away. If you can't travel to an expert, ask your doctor if she has computer contact with anyone who is expert in the field. It's a growing trend, and many doctors will be willing to contact the expert—and also be willing to learn about the subject.

It's vital that you have a doctor who you can

Cut out all caffeine from your diet.

trust, and who will trust you. Many cases of RLS are mild and simple, and one or two medications can be prescribed for use during attacks. Other cases of RLS are severe and keep people from working and from having anything like a normal life. These are the ones who need all the help they can find. A doctor should be available at any time to prescribe new drugs, or to adjust those being used to meet the varying demands of the disease.

UNDERLYING FACTORS

Most physicians will check with patient's overall health before moving on to medications. There are several factors that can bring on or make your RLS worse. The doctor will have a frank discussion with you about these.

One is caffeine. If you drink a lot of coffee, or down four to six cans of soft drinks with caffeine in them each day, your doctor will advise you to eliminate all caffeine from your diet. Simply cutting out caffeine in all of its products—such as soft drinks, tea, coffee, chocolate, and hot cocoa—can bring a sudden halt to RLS symptoms in some people. Even if it is not the primary cause, caffeine will make any RLS worse than if you don't use caffeine. So, big signpost: **Cut out all caffeine from your diet.**

While we're talking about drinking, the use of alcohol deserves some equal time. Some people continue to use alcohol to help them get to sleep at night. They drink themselves into a stupor and nod off. For some it works, but only for the first half of the night. After that the insomnia usually returns—ruining the rest of the night's sleep. For some people insomnia is what causes them to start abusing alcohol.

ALTERNATIVE TREATMENTS FOR RLS

So far, a single cause for RLS has not been found. Until that happens there can be no guaranteed

A five minute stretching workout can do wonders.

cure for the disease. Which leaves us in that in-between when miracle cures blossom for a short time and then wither and vanish. Or when some report a total remission or cure of RLS only to have it slam back and be worse than ever, months or years later.

While there are no known cures for RLS, over the years some treatments have proved to be effective for some patients in lessening the intensity of the RLS symptoms. These include some of the following techniques.

NEUROMUSCULAR MASSAGE THERAPY

Deep muscle massage can help a patient who has worked her legs too hard or too long. Some patients ride a bike too long, or take hikes that are counterproductive. From this overuse, blood vessels and nerves can be trapped in hardened muscles. Unless that pressure is relieved, localized inflow of arterial blood can result. This is big trouble.

Deep massage can help relieve that problem. Often this type of massage is painful, but in this case no pain, no gain—and the rewards are gratifying. Before going to a massage therapist, be sure you know what training they have had and what type of deep massage they will use. Some therapists say that patients can do a lot themselves to help their situation. They say that a five minute stretching workout in the morning can do wonders. Patients should also be careful of what and how they eat. Therapists say that it is indeed beneficial to gently massage an area of the body that hurts, because muscles are like sponges. You can squeeze out toxins such as lactic acid.

While we're talking about massage, this is a good place to say that using a mechanical or electrical vibrator can be helpful in relieving RLS symptoms. There are some reports on this in current medical literature.

Acupressure point

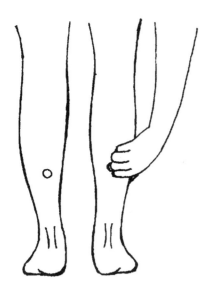

While sitting, press with thumbs or squeeze the center of the base of your calf muscles. Hold for one minute.

SCLEROTHERAPY

This is an old non-surgical method of eliminating varicose veins. Intravenous injections of a solution are made directly into the affected veins. This starts an inflammatory response that shrinks and eventually leads to the reabsorption of the vein. This treatment is done during several sessions as an outpatient. It sometimes involves the use of ultrasound to guide deeper injections for invisible veins.

Some authorities say that correctly fitted support hose can help alleviate symptoms of venous insufficiency. It may be that RLS and leg vein diseases have a common connection. So wearing support hose may help give relief to some RLS patients.

Be careful. Non-prescription over-the-counter support hose may cause more harm than help. High quality support hose—sometimes known as surgical or post-operative weight hose—are usually obtained only by prescription after a custom fitting. They come in 20-30 or 30-40 graduated strength.

Do you have troublesome varicose veins? The bulging, blue kind are easy to see, but the sub-surface ones are harder to locate. There aren't a lot of specialists who know about varicose veins in the doctor population. It may be harder to find one than it is to find a doctor who knows about RLS. The hunt for a good vein specialist may be worth the trouble.

VITAMINS, HERBS AND DIETS

VITAMIN E

Not a lot of medical literature to back up any concrete results, but one doctor reported that he had used 400 IU vitamin E capsules three times a day on a patient for a dermatological condition. The patient also had RLS, and she reported a cessation of the "jumping leg" problem. The same doctor said he had seen such results with nine of his skin ailment patients.

> There aren't a lot of specialists who know about varicose veins.

25

Folic Acid of the Vitamin B Complex

One researcher said that he believed that the folic acid shortage in pregnant women could make the RLS worse. He said a test showed that 60% of senior citizens had folic acid levels below normal, and many of them had RLS.

Folate can be found in beet greens, kale, leafy green vegetables, and spinach. Liver and kidneys also provide good amounts of the nutrient. A caution here. Over-cooking destroys most of the folate, especially in vegetables. Steaming is suggested.

A recent study shows that RLS patients respond well to sizeable doses of folic acid—up to 10 mg per day.

Iron

Most multi-vitamin/mineral supplements these days include iron in the mixture. Everyone should be encouraged to take daily multi-vitamin and mineral supplements. Any deficiency in iron in the system is thought to be a culprit in the intensity of the RLS. Iron-deficient anemia has long been tied with RLS. Some arthritis drugs may tend to eliminate or cut down on the level of iron in the body. Check with your doctor to be sure the iron level in your bloodstream is adequate.

Magnesium

Recently, researchers have reported that many RLS patients are deficient in magnesium. You might check your magnesium level with your doctor. This mineral is also beneficial in other ways, and it could help your RLS.

Aromatic Herbs

Some people say that the use of aromatic herbs can be of help in getting to sleep even during RLS attacks. They say that clary sage and ylang ylang can help ease depression, and alleviate anger. To lessen mental stress, anxiety and nervousness, try Chamo-

Clary sage and Ylang Ylang can help ease depression.

mile and lavender. Put them under the edge of the pillow slip next to your head. Remember, these aromatic herbs are meant to aid rest by their scent alone and are not to be taken internally in this case.

CORRECT EXERCISE CAN HELP

After an hour of twisting, kicking, turning over and stretching out, nothing will ease your restless legs this night, so you get out of bed and start walking through the house, then you begin marching in place. Many times the problem persists—the creepy crawly feeling won't go away.

Sometimes RLS patients punish their legs trying to get rid of the restless feelings. Often it works the other way, and needed blood has a hard time getting through knotted muscles and hardened tissue to perform its duty.

Yes, your prescription medications are going to help—as well as warm soaking tub baths and massage. The idea is to get those muscles relaxed and softened so blood can work through the tissue and do its healing work.

There are also some simple stretching exercises that can help. Yes, you need to get out of bed and do your thing on the exercise bike, or the stair climber or just walk around your house, but first you should do some stretching. Every sport has a warm up procedure before the game. Watch the NFL football warm ups before games. Even baseball players have routines of pre-play exercises and stretching. There are good reasons for this.

Try these stretching exercises every day, and especially some of them before your night walking. One note here. For any exercise that calls for you to lie on the floor, you usually can do the same thing on your bed. The older you get, the harder it will be to get up off the floor. (An eighty-year-old made this suggestion and it is a good one.)

Exercises where you lie on your back can be done on your bed or the floor.

1. Lie on the floor or your bed on your back. Lift both legs upward to a 90-degree position, keeping knees straight. Now put your hands on the inside of your thighs and push your legs outward. Hold for thirty seconds, then move hands to outside of thighs and push legs back together. Repeat this stretch eight times, bringing legs back to the floor after each stretch.

2. Sit on the floor, placing your back against a wall. Put the loop of a hand towel around your foot's arch. Holding the towel ends with both hands, lift your leg upward, keeping your knee straight. This will stretch the back of your leg muscles. Bring it as high as you can, then gently lower to the floor. Do this stretch with regular breathing. Repeat fifteen times.

3. Sit on the floor. Bend one leg to the side and extend the other one straight in front. Hold your ankle or foot of the extended leg with both hands. Now slowly bend forward at the waist as far as you can go, stretching back and leg muscles. Increase this stretch gradually until you become flexible enough to bring your head almost to your leg. Hold this position for twenty seconds. Repeat five times. Then do the same thing with the other leg.

4. Squat on the floor and put both hands on the floor in front. Then stretch out your right leg behind you as far as you can, resting it on your toes. Hold this position for ten seconds. Bring your right leg

back and extend your left leg in the same stretch. Repeat with both legs ten times.

5. Stand near a wall, and lean against it with your arms straight, hands flat on the wall. You may need to move your feet forward or back to get in this position. Now gradually work your feet backward until you can feel the tendons stretching and straining in the back of your leg and ankle. Keep your feet flat on the floor. Stretch the tendons more by bending your arms a little and leaning farther forward. Hold this position for 20 seconds, then relax and shake out your legs. Repeat five times.

6. Lie on your back on the floor or your bed, lift your knees up and put them together. Then with your hands, push your knees from side to side without using your leg muscles. This helps move the outer and inner thigh muscles. Repeat ten times.

Exercise morning, noon or night, but do it!

MORE LEG STRETCHING EXERCISES

Try these when you get up, at noon, afternoon, and especially when you have restless legs and want to get up and run around. The exercising can sometimes help. Several times a day won't hurt.

7. Standing barefoot at a counter or dresser, with feet a foot apart. Put hands flat on the counter and lift up on your toes as high as you can, raising your heels off the floor. Hold for five seconds, then lower slowly to the floor. Do this one ten times.

8. Same position as #7, but with your toes pointing to the sides. Now squat gently.

This is different from deep knee bends. Works different muscles. Feel the muscles on the inner side of thighs and legs stretch. Do this ten times.

9. At the same counter, turn sideways, hold with one hand and extend one leg all the way forward and upward until it's even with your waist. Try pointing your toe. Do ten times. Then do the same leg extending to the rear ten times. Repeat on second leg.

10. At the same counter, holding with one hand and standing sideways, lift your knee straight up as high as you can—waist level or higher. Hold for three counts, then lower. Repeat ten times. Then do the same leg, kicking your heel toward your buttocks and hold for three seconds. Do ten times. Now do the other leg the same way.

Try some of these, and use the ones that fit you best.

If you like to exercise in the water, most large cities have exercise groups at city pools or YMCAs or YWCAs. Look around, you'll find one. Water supports part of the body weight and makes exercising easier.

Additional acupressure point

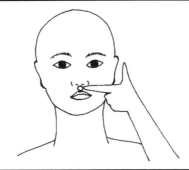

Press with index finger or knuckle in the groove between your nose and upper lip. Hold for one minute while breathing deeply.

MEDICAL TREATMENTS FOR RLS

If your doctor is well founded in RLS, he or she will do the testing and take your history and then decide if your RLS is severe enough to require medication. It may be that together you will find that some of the alternative means detailed in the previous chapter will be enough to treat your RLS.

If together you decide that the steps taken already do not do the job, then you should talk about medications. If you decide that the RLS has harmed your quality of life and that nothing else you do can keep it in control, then you'll need to move on to medications.

Your case may be one that will not need medication every day to control the night-time leg kicking. Let's say you get along well, except on long bus or train or plane trips, or at long parties where you can't get up and move around. For occasional use,

"PRN" means the patient can take the medicine when needed.

31

your doctor may prescribe a "prn" medication. This medical shorthand stands for the patient using the prescription pills only when needed.

When you and your doctor agree that your RLS is bad enough that it happens most days and sometimes most nights as well, you probably will be given drugs to take on a daily basis.

Most doctors will select the drug they think will work and prescribe it in a small dose to see the effect. They will monitor the patient closely to watch for side effects. Gradually the size of the dose will be increased until the RLS is controlled. If there are no side effects that are severe enough to go to another drug, this one will be standardized for this patient.

Sometimes an RLS patient will need a dosage higher than is generally recommended. This is a case where the patient and the doctor must agree. If the patient needs the higher dose and it works, usually the doctor will agree to it. The patient is the most important one here.

Well before the doctor and patient agree on a medication, there should be a complete history of the patient—including any drugs that he or she is now taking for other problems or illnesses. Some drugs conflict with other drugs. Some can negate the second one. Sometimes the combination of drugs can be fatal.

For this reason most pharmacies now will keep a history of regular patients in their computer and, when a new drug is prescribed, they will check the computer and see if there is any conflict or problem with other drugs the patient is now using.

This would be a great idea for doctors to do as well, but most as of yet don't have the computer capacity to keep all of their patients' history in their hard drive. They should.

If the medication the doctor gives you does not work, or if it has too many side effects, you'll need a different medication. Not all drugs work the same on

Take RLS medication a half hour before symptoms occur.

all people. For that reason the doctor has a group of drugs that usually work, and he'll start using the next one he thinks might do the job.

If one drug doesn't seem to be working, the doctor may want to give you a combination of drugs. Together they might control the RLS and at the same time not have the bad side effects.

Sometimes your doctor will use what is called symptomatic therapy. This might be when one physical condition is causing or greatly magnifying your RLS. An example would be low iron in your blood. For this the doctor would simply put you on iron pills and monitor your blood iron level until it is at the right point.

The same would then be done for any other physical problem, using drugs when needed.

Medications for an RLS patient should be taken to anticipate the symptom. For example if your leg problems begin as soon as you go to bed, you should take medications for that problem a half hour before you hit the sack. For some medications, the time they activate may be up to an hour later, so know from your doctor how long the medication takes to function and act accordingly for any of your RLS medications.

Sometimes medications will wear off after four or five hours, depending on the type. If you take one at bed time for your legs and it works fine until five hours later, you may need to take another dose at that time so you can get back to sleep in a half hour. If your symptoms are bad during the day, you may need to take that medication several times during the day to keep the pain and the problem under control.

Sometimes a doctor will want to rotate your medication. Say you have one that works well for your RLS problem and has few side effects. After three or four weeks, your body may start to adjust to the medication and it may not be as effective. If this happens your doctor will rotate you to a new medica-

There are four classifications of RLS medicines.

tion for several weeks. Then you might go back to the first one. It doesn't happen often, but if it happens to you, you need to know about rotation of medications. Some medications should not be stopped abruptly. This can cause serious problems. If you do rotate drugs, be sure that the doctor has you taper off your dosage for a week or so before you start the new system.

WHAT MEDICATIONS WORK ON RLS?

We'll look at four classifications of drugs here:

1. **Medications most likely to help RLS patients.**

2. **Those which may be worth a try, but have not been studied as much, or used as successfully as those in the first group.**

3. **Symptomatic medications aimed at particular triggers of RLS.**

4. **Medications that RLS patients should avoid.**

A brief note of warning: Medications of all types for all kinds of diseases and illnesses are on a cutting edge. New ones come out every few months. Older ones are changed and are used for new purposes. Three or four years can make a huge difference in what drugs and medications are used for any disease—including RLS as well. So be sure to check with your doctor and your pharmacist to see that the drugs mentioned here are still in favor, and to find out about new ones that can be used when you are reading this.

1. DRUGS FOR BASIC RLS TREATMENT

These are the drugs that most doctors prescribe for RLS because of double blind studies and practical experience. They have been found to work for all or most RLS patients.

BENZODIAZEPINES

These are sedating type drugs and are used to treat RLS and PLMS. One of these drugs is Valium, which has been used for RLS since the sixties. One basic advantage of the benzodiazepines is that they are safer than some other drugs. They can cause drowsiness and even stupor if overdosed, but there is little chance of a fatal dose.

The strong point of these drugs is that they can increase the quality of sleep. They also can be helpful to reduce incidence of waking RLS, but this is less well documented.

The most used drug of this type is Klonopin, which is usually taken at bedtime. This drug also helps in other sleep disorders such as Sleep Behavior Disorder, where patients act out their dreams and sometimes jump out of bed or strike their bed mate.

Doses for various benzodiazepines are:

Klonopin, doses of .05 to 2 mg.
Restoril, doses of 15 to 45 mg.
Halcion, doses of 0.125 to 5 mg.
Valium (daytime use), dose of 5 mg twice a day.

DOPAMINERGIC AGENTS

Drugs of this type work on the dopamine system of the central nervous system. The central nervous system includes the spinal cord within the spine and the brain within the skull. Dopamine is one of the neurotransmitters that are used by nerve cells to communicate with each other. This system of communication through the brain and spinal cord is believed to be important to RLS but researchers are not sure just how it works.

Typical doses of L-DOPA are 10/100 to 100/400 mg. These doses are usually taken at bedtime. One problem is that when they wear off there can be a rebound of the symptoms. Side effects here can be

> **Dopamine is one of the neurotransmitters in your brain.**

35

stomach discomfort, nausea and vomiting, and head-
ache. If the medication is the sustained release type, it
should be taken one-and-a-half hours before bedtime.
These L-DOPA drugs can be taken during the day
as well, but if round-the-clock medication is
needed, then some other type should be tried. L-
DOPA can be used as a "prn" medication—used by
the patient when needed.

OPIOIDS

Opioids are man-made compounds that act
much like natural opiates. These chemicals all induce
sedation or sleep, and are called narcotic. It is thought
that these opioids work through the endogenous
opiate system. Some researchers say that the opioids may work through the dopamine system. They
all are helpful in treating RLS, and probably for
PLMS as well.

Many different opioid medications have been
used on RLS including Davon, Percodan, Talwin and
methadone. Doses vary but can be: codeine, 15 to 240
mg daily; Darvon, 130 to 520 mg a day; Percodan, 2.5
to 20 mg per day; Talwin, 50 to 200 mg per day;
methadone, 5 to 30 mg per day.

Opioids are taken just before symptoms are
expected—in the evening, at night or during the day.
They can be taken on a prn basis.

The major worry about using narcotics is addiction. However, addiction is rare in RLS patients, since
they use the narcotic drug less than with some
other diseases.

Another drug much used is a dopamine precur-
sor, Sinemet.

The usual dose is 300 mg a day. Some doctors
say that Sinemet use will result in the need for higher
and higher doses to achieve the same result. Some
patients say they feel like a "junkie" because they
depend on that dose twice or more a day.

2. SECONDARY TREATMENT DRUGS

These are medications that have not had long-term successful use with RLS. Most of these medical compounds may have special uses, but most doctors seem to go to them only after the primary drugs shown above do not give satisfactory results.

ANTICONVULSANT MEDICATIONS

Anticonvulsant compounds are used to stop seizures. They are used mainly for epilepsy, and for seizures before or during strokes, and other situations where seizures are present. Some of these medications are reported to be helpful for RLS patients. These include Tegretol, Depakene, and Neurontin. Not enough research has been done on these medications, and it is not known how they work on the body—however, in some instances they have been beneficial.

Doses have been shown as: Tegretol 600 to 1200 mg per day, Depakene 1000 to 3000 mg per day, and Neurontin 300 to 2700 mg per day. There are some dangers with these drugs, and they may cause injuries to the white blood cells and liver, so blood monitoring must be done twice a year on patients taking these medications.

MEDICATIONS DEALING WITH THE ADRENERGIC SYSTEM

The adrenergic system is made up of cells whose neurotransmitters are adrenaline and noradrenaline. These cells in effect "tune up" the brain. Catapres is a medication which is an alpha receptor antagonist, and is helpful in many RLS patients, especially for restlessness.

Doses have been shown as 0.3 to 0.7 milligrams. Some patients need to have higher doses.

The use of Catapres therapy needs to be done gradually, starting with 0.1 mg at night. This is because the drug may bring about a steep drop in blood pressure. No one with a low blood pressure

Abrupt discontinuance of Inderal can cause serious heart damage.

37

problem should use Catapres.

Inderal, a beta receptor blocker, has been reported by some medical authorities to help with RLS. The dose is not firmly established, but ranges from 40 to 320 mg per day. Treatment must be started gradually, usually with a 10 mg pill, and must never be discontinued suddenly. Abrupt discontinuance of Inderal can result in serious heart damage.

3. TRIGGER-SPECIFIC MEDICATIONS

MIRAPEX

This drug is usually only prescribed for someone who has moderate to severe RLS and for whom other treatments didn't work. Most reports on Mirapex are good. It should be started with a small dose, increasing as needed until the symptoms are relieved.

One side effect here can be insomnia, even though it might totally resolve the RLS symptoms. To counter this, the medication can be taken during the day, with the last one about 5 p.m. Usually this medication is not taken on an empty stomach. Between meals use a banana or crackers or some ginger tea. Be careful driving or operating machinery if you take Mirapex. There have been some problems in this area. Dosage usually is .125 to 1.5 mg a day.

BACLOFEN

This medication is for Multiple Sclerosis patients who also have Periodic Limb Movement Syndrome. The drug has been tested, and tends to reduce the intensity but not the frequency of the movements. It is reported that Baclofen also helps some RLS patients.

4. MEDICATIONS FOR THE RLS PATIENT TO AVOID

Neuroleptics, which are used to treat serious psychiatric disorders, should not be taken by RLS

Caffeine is on the avoidance list for RLS patients.

38

patients. They act to reduce the activity of the dopamine system of the brain. This is bad for RLS patients, since they need medications that can increase this dopamine activity. These medications include Thorazine, Haldol and Mellaril. These meds can also cause restlessness, which can appear to be just like RLS restlessness.

Reglan is another drug that RLS patients should avoid. It is normally used to prevent stomach irritation.

Caffeine, while not a medication, is on the avoidance list for RLS patients. Most doctors say that the reduction or elimination of caffeine should be a first step in RLS treatment.

Most antidepressants should be avoided by RLS patients. Talk to your doctor. Don't suddenly stop taking an antidepressant your doctor has prescribed. She might not know you also have RLS.

Most of the tricyclics such as Anafranil, Ascendin, Etrafon and Elavil—and many others—will worsen your RLS symptoms.

If you have depression and RLS, your doctor might work with drugs such as Desyrel, Remeron or Serzone, but even these must be used with caution.

Antihistamines, especially Benadryl, can aggravate RLS symptoms. Many over-the-counter medications for colds, hay fever and sinus contain diphenhydramine. This is in Excedrin PM, Tylenol PM and Bayer. Even the seasick pills, Dramamine, have this chemical. In some cases RLS patients say Benadryl helps them sleep. For others it keeps them awake. See which works for you.

ANTI-NAUSEA DRUGS

Most of these drugs used in the U.S. are dopamine antagonists. They decrease the availability of dopamine and can seriously exacerbate the RLS symptoms. Some of these are Antivert, Atarax,

To Sinemet or not to Sinemet?

Compazine, and Phenergan. Consult your health care provider for one of the newer, and much more expensive drugs, that RLS patients can take with safety.

SINEMET

This drug has been suggested in a previous section as one that will work to lower the intensity of RLS symptoms. Some patients and doctors disagree. One says he has a survey that shows that six out of seven patients who use Sinemet wind up with worse symptoms as Sinemet wears off. They say that they need more and more Sinemet to do the job. They become junkies waiting for their next "fix" to ward off the RLS symptoms.

Other RLS patients swear by—not at—Sinemet, saying they have little rebound and that it overall is a helpful drug for them to take and they are happy with it. See how it works for you.

COPING WITH RLS

So, you have RLS. You've been to the doctor, you're taking all of the precautions and doing the exercises and taking the hot baths and doing everything the support group suggested, but still you have the restlessness, the getting up at night, the night walking. Just how do you program yourself and your family to cope with, to live with RLS?

One woman said living with RLS is like making love to an alligator—it must be done with extreme care.

True.

So, how does your RLS affect your life? Your bed is more than just a place to sleep. It's also the platform for your lovemaking.

"Not tonight, dear, I'm just too tired." This is going to work a few times, but unless your spouse is attuned to your special RLS life, it isn't going to work for long.

Yes, you are tired. You've been in agony half the

> **Making love stops all RLS pain and problems— for about ten minutes.**

41

day, then in the evening you couldn't sit still to watch the regular TV shows, and then when you slipped into bed, the first thing you felt were those creepy-crawly critters attacking your legs. You had to get up and walk into the living room and back a few times or you would explode!

So when you get back, your husband is flaked out on the bed dead to the world and he won't wake up until the alarm goes off in seven hours. You stare at him a minute. So do you get in bed, wake him up, give it a try, and probably disappoint him with your performance because you're beat—or let him sleep? Usually you let him sleep and you grab a pillow and blanket and steal into the living room and curl up on the couch—until your legs drive you crazy again.

Or you do give in and try to be quiet and passionate. It goes well or not well and when it's over nobody is satisfied. One wag said that making love for an RLS person stopped all of the pain and the leg problems—for about ten minutes.

For RLS patients on the right medications, the bed becomes less of a fighting field, and often sleep can come in four-hour chunks—then hopefully more. Medications and life style changes can make the huge difference here.

OTHER PROBLEMS

Ever thought about having to stand up to finish a meal in a restaurant? Or of getting up twice during the same meal to go to the bathroom just so you can walk a little bit to relieve the pain and creepy-crawly feeling in your legs? Happens to RLS patients.

Coping with going to a movie or a concert or even church can be a trial. In case of a sudden flare-up of jittery leg muscles, you'll want to be sure that you have an aisle seat. Otherwise it develops into a climb over legs, over skirts and trousers, and a thousand pardon-me apologies. An idea: In most live

Try standing room tickets at your next theatre outing.

theatres they have what they call standing room tickets. They usually cost less as well. Most RLS patients will be glad to stand up during a two-hour show. It makes it immediate and simple to do a little walk even during the performance to calm legs or to get the muscles tuned up again.

Taking a trip? Going by car is best, but have someone else drive. Then you can stop every half-hour if you have to, should a rough day of attacks from RLS have you on the ropes. Be sure your spouse, or other driver, understands your situation—it makes those stops and little walks easier all the way around. A train can also be a workable idea. Plenty of room to walk up and down the aisles, go from car to car. Worse is a plane. True it takes less time, but a five-hour flight is still five hours, no matter how many miles you cross. If you must fly, tell the flight attendants your situation, and that sometimes you simply have to get up and walk the narrow aisles. They will understand and help all they can.

A bus trip is probably the worst way to travel. Slow and almost no room to walk—even if the driver will let you (for safety reasons). Stay away from the bus.

TRY NOT TO PANIC

It's late at night. You have been rousted out of bed by jittery leg muscles and they won't let you lie down without setting off again. You have trouble sitting. You tried a hot tub and that did nothing for you. More and more you're feeling angry and tired and stressed and picked on. Why you? Why do you have to be so tired but not able to sleep? So ready to lie down but not able to? Quietly the idea of suicide may slip into your mind and mightn't go away.

Many RLS patients in this situation grab the phone and call someone. Best if you have a digital phone or one that you can walk around with that has a base radio connection. Walk and talk. Call another RLS patient if you know one. Chances are they might be up doing the night walk with you. Even if not, they won't mind talking with you and keeping up your spirits for a while. It often can be a tremendous help just knowing that someone else is in the same situation that you are.

Even though talking with someone else about the anguish of a sudden attack of RLS can help, it's still up to you to take control and command of the situation. Here are the Golden Rules Of Coping with Panic that Ann Landers used in her column several years ago. They certainly apply to RLS people as well. Check them out:

Change your "what if" thinking.

1. **Remember that though the feelings and symptoms you are experiencing are frightening, they are neither dangerous nor life threatening. Take time to take ten deep breaths, as deep as you can make them and hold them as long as you can before exhaling. This will increase the oxygen supply to your brain and your whole body.**

2. **Know that what you are experiencing is merely an exaggeration of normal reactions to stress. Your heart may beat a bit faster and that is indeed normal, the old "run from danger" adrenal rush.**

3. **Remember, fighting the feelings that you might explode or trying to wish the crawlies away are futile. Recognize the fact that your need to move about is real, physical and temporary. You know it does go away, maybe a bit slower than you'd like, but it does go away in time.**

4. **Yes, there will be an end to your legs**

44

misery. You may be one of those who are affected by changes in the weather. This is not considered scientific, but many RLS patients find their legs respond negatively to the rise and fall of the barometer. Listen to the weather report. There may be a storm near you. You can't do anything about the weather. Remember, every time the barometer falls, it rises again.

5. Don't dwell on your fear that this might get worse. Stay in the present and be aware of what is happening to you, and think of ways to relieve your pain and insistent need to walk around.

6. Count your uneasiness level from zero to ten and watch it go up and down. Notice that it doesn't stay at level ten for more than a few seconds.

7. Change your "what if" thinking. Think of something to do. Work on your computer, or the garden. Stand up at the kitchen counter and play solitaire. Get at the ironing you've put off for weeks. Do any simple task that you can perform even if you have to jump and down while you do it. Keeping the brain active seems to help the anxiety wear itself out.

8. Be aware of the moment when you stop thinking frightening thoughts and peace begins to creep over your body.

9. Wait and let the quiet enfold you. Don't be in a hurry. Think about how good you will feel when the anxiety and jumpiness have passed completely.

10. Think of how much better you feel than

you did hours ago. Relish that moment of peace when you are in total control. It's time to go back to work or back to bed.

FAMILY NEEDS

If you have a family, or just a spouse, it is vital for you to remember that they have needs too. Always try to put your medications and your rituals for relief in a form—and with timing—that allows you to handle the needed chores and work around the home. Make time to get the kids off to school or to get your spouse's dinner when you both come home from work or play.

There are ways to do this. Organize. Try to do certain things around the house once a week instead of daily. You probably need to vacuum only once a week. Do cleaning on only one day. Allow plenty of time to rest and to do your medications.

Remember to take your pills on time. Don't skip pills. Make out a chart and have a week-long pill holder that keeps your pills at hand and ready to take. Work your medication chart. Remember that some night time medications have a three-hour life span. Most medications take about a half- hour to dissolve and get into the system to do their job. Which means a ten p.m. pill will work from ten-thirty until one-thirty a.m. Another pill might be needed to get you through the night.

CAN YOU HAVE RLS AND STILL HOLD A JOB?

The easy answer is yes and no. If your RLS is mild and bothers you little during the day, you probably will have no trouble holding most any kind of job you can do.

On the other hand, if you regularly need medication during the day for leg tremors or jitters, if you can't stand to sit for more than ten minutes at a

Get a daily use pill holder for the week's pills.

time, if you must have a walk around every hour or so, you will probably will have trouble keeping a traditional job. The first thing to do is talk to your remarkably understanding boss and work out a job you can do and the times you need off to medicate.

If you have three or four nights in a row that you get no sleep, you are going to be ineffective in almost any kind of day job. If it's a dangerous job, you could get somebody injured or killed. You might even be the casualty yourself.

The ideal job for anyone with RLS is to be self-employed. Then you can adjust your work load to your state of health. On bad days you don't get any work done. On good days you do more than you normally would. You might even start working nights if that is possible in your own business, to keep things humming.

Few people with RLS have the chance to run their own business. In fact many of the RLS patients are in their fifties and sixties and many are retired, so the work problem is not theirs.

For those who must work, RLS is a problem. First take stock of your physical ability. If the RLS is a recent onset, make sure of what you can do now, then go talk with your supervisor or your boss. Demonstrate what you can and can't do. Request a new job—or change in responsibility—which meets your physical abilities. Many employers will work with a handicapped person. Indeed there is a new law that mandates that employers must adjust work schedules and jobs to match a handicapped person's abilities. You might need to remind your supervisor or employer about this law.

If you have a job and have an onset of RLS, get to your doctor at once and try to find medications that will let you get enough sleep at night so you can work. Then try to adjust your job and your hours of work, so you can get through the day and

Show your boss what you can do on the job.

be productive.

Half the secret here is to get the right medication so you can get enough sleep, then talk with your employer about your situation. Devise a way you can stay on the job, be productive for the company, and still fight off as many of the effects of RLS as you can with medications, life style changes, diet and anything else that will help.

JOIN AN RLS SUPPORT GROUP

There is nothing more comforting to an individual in pain than to talk to someone who is "wearing her shoes"—who knows the battle and has been through the fire of the situation.

That's why if you now have RLS and do not belong to a support group, you should find one. If there is not one in your area, start one. We'll show you how later on.

Support groups are sprouting up all over the map. The first ones most of us remember were Alcoholics Anonymous. Since then there have been support groups for drugs and smoking and gambling and for almost every disease known to mankind. There may be one in your area for RLS, and if you can't find one, we'll show you how to check it out with the experts.

What happens at a support group? It's a meeting in someone's home or in a hospital or public meeting room where people get together, weekly or every two

With a support group, you don't have to feel you're alone.

weeks, and talk about their pains and their victories in the fight against RLS. Usually there is no "director," no professional—it's a one-on-one, I'll tell you my story if you tell me yours. Groups operate in all sorts of ways. Some allow an hour for testimonials and individual's stories about what is happening to them and how they are trying to stop the pain and sleeplessness.

Some then have speakers. This might be a physician who specializes in RLS. It might be a nurse or some specialists in coping with RLS who can give the group some good advice and some encouragement—and most of all fire up in them the will to keep on battling.

Some RLS groups have refreshments; some have only decaf coffee or tea and ice water or soft drinks. Sometimes they last for only an hour. Sometimes there are breaks every fifteen minutes for everyone to get up and move around to get rid of the "jitters" and the "creepy crawly" feelings. Look at fifty RLS support groups and you'll find fifty different routines, rituals, methods and times and places of meeting.

The time, place and operation aren't important—it's the interchange, the networking, the sharing of experiences and knowing that you are not alone out there at 3 a.m. when you need to call somebody to talk it through. Just that contact often is enough to make the support group worthwhile.

One of the big benefits of belonging to a support group is to find out that others with the same problem are getting help. If they can, you can too. It gives you a lift and a new way to look at things.

Medications come in for a lot of talk at these meetings. What works for one won't work for someone else. But if it does work for that person, it might be worth a try for you. You make a note of the name and call your doctor the next morning.

On the most basic level, attending a support

group for RLS gives you the wonderful knowledge that there are others out there who suffer the same way you do. Who have the aches and the night walks and the small and large panics that affect you. Just knowing that you aren't alone is one of the marvelous experiences of going to your first RLS meeting.

Doctors will be a major topic of conversation. Some might say that there are only a handful of doctors in this area who have even heard of RLS. Others might simply say don't go to doctor so and so, because he gave me Advil and told me to go home and do something about my wild imagination. Others will tout their own doctors, saying that they couldn't be nicer and more sympathetic and that they really know what RLS is and have treated dozens of patients.

Often there are printed handouts for all who attend. These might come from a national organization called the Restless Legs Syndrome Foundation. We'll talk more about it later. You can use these handouts to read up on RLS and, when you fully understand the material, you can pass it on to your doctor who may not be as up-to-date on RLS as you are.

A support group can help you find a good RLS doctor.

NATIONWIDE SUPPORT GROUPS

If you're really serious about joining a support group, there is an easy way to see if there is already one in your area. Just keep reading. The RLS Foundation has a web site, which lists most of the RLS support groups in the United States and abroad.

In case you don't have a computer or aren't on the Internet, here is a printout of the sites. Remember these will change. For the very latest information, punch up the RLS web site at **www.rls.org** and scroll down and click on "support groups" for the latest names and phone numbers and email addresses.

Here they are:

ALABAMA:
Shoals Area:
  Coretha Downs, 256-247-3171
  Maxine Crouch, 205-446-5311, jtassoc@hiwaay.net
ARIZONA:
Scottsdale:
  Lynne Gessner, 480-9470-0009
  Joan Schebler, 480-949-9918, 1gess@doitnow.com
NW Valley:
  Loretta DeSandro, 623-584-5608, lordes@inficad.com
  Marilyn Butterfield, 623-566-2653, MGB956l@hotmail.com
ARKANSAS:
Hot Springs Village:
  Enid Scripture, 501-922-0049, escriptu@msn.com
CALIFORNIA:
San Francisco Peninsula:
  Gretchen Smithey, 650-401-8026
  Joanne Bellan, 415-664-2366
San Francisco East Bay:
  Dori Davi, 510-837-7711
Orange County:
  Hetty Olwin, 714-962-0578.
Central Coast:
  Sue Arzouman, 805-534-0734, jimsuearzouman@email.msn.com
San Diego:
  Sharon Burley, 619-558-7681, sburley@webtv.net
Oceanside:
  Jeanette Speake, 760-940-0487
  Lou Engel, 760-439-4093
Inland Empire:
  Grace Ruggles, 909-887-3732
  Mary Petri, 909-792-1794
Southern California:
  Elizabeth L. Tunison, 562-699-4917, tuni22@aol.com
  Southern California RLS website, www.come.to/rls
COLORADO:
Denver:
  June Sheridan, 303-344-4964
  Marge Fuhr, 303-494-4913, DDFuhr@aol.com

CONNECTICUT:

Cyberspace:

Jodi Judson, jmjudson@nettaxi.com

Cyberspace Support Group website, www.mlists.net/judson/rls.html

Southern Connecticut:

Patty Yurkas, 203-327-5729 Yurkas@ibm.net

Reggie Springer, 203-324-5733, Rcs4pas@aol.com

DELAWARE:

Eastern Shores:

Micki Buck, 410-749-5911

Bonnie Wise, 410-208-2810.

Broward County:

Lillian Kaufman, 945-724-0438, Lillian00@webtv.net

FLORIDA:

Central Florida:

Barbara Stock, 407-629-8791: brstock@aol.com

Lower Pinellas County:

Virginia G. England, 813-518-6200, v.g.england@juno.com

Palm Coast:

Charlotte M. Schultz, 904-445-7158: schatzie@pcfl.net

South Florida:

Jeanne Kalish, 561-495-1555

Joy Kahn, 561-488-4557, Joyb222@aol.com

Sarasota/Manatee:

Thelma Bradt, 941-359-6389: tbradt@mindspring.com

GEORGIA:

Atlanta:

Dick Hawkins, 770-938-4709, klihawk@mindspring.com

ILLINOIS:

Southern Illinois

Linda Patterson, 618-826-4260, paterson@midwest.net

Northern Illinois:

Nancy Yang, 847-244-0180, Nancyy2@aol.com

INDIANA:

1st Indy RLS/PLMD:

Andriene Egger, 317-578-8146, adrienej.egger@worldnet.att.net

IOWA:

Central Iowa:

Delila Roberts, 515-597-2782

Elaine Tucker, 515-388-4736.

KANSAS:

Eastern Kansas:

Barbara Wacker, 913-682-4537, bwcol@lvnworth.com

MAINE:

Restless In Maine:

Karlene Fenderson, 207-777-8580, karlene@exploremaine.com

Theodore Beaudoin, 207-783-3151

MARYLAND:

Baltimore Area:

Patricia Sarratt, 410-879-6943, srrtt@yahoo.com

Beatrice Weitzel, 410-254-4456

MASSACHUSETTS:

All Massachusetts:

Sheila Connolly, 508-790-7640, Sfconnolly@capecod.net

Carol Connolly, 781-641-1104, carol.connolly@simmons.edu

MICHIGAN:

SE Michigan:

Lillian Eory, 734-641-1135: elolrly1@aol.com

Oakland County:

Shelly Skelton, 248-682-7228: shelskel@juno.com

Western Michigan:

Neva Warsen, 616-532-1698: nmwarsen@aol.com

MINNESOTA:

SW Minnesota Walkers:

Rosewitha Seltz, 320-857-7047, Scountry@hutchtel.net

MISSOURI:

St. Louis:

Hanne Spence, 314-487-0370, Hmspence@artsci.wustl.edu

NEBRASKA:

Greater Omaha:

Linda Sieh, 402-832-5321, lorensieh@hotmail.com

Joan Sulentic, 712-566-2668.

Southeast Nebraska:

Connie Clark, 402-474-5632, cowboy@inebraska.com

NEVADA:

Southern Nevada:

Leeann & John Felbaum, 702-294-0540,
SouthernNevadaRLS@hotmail.com

NEW HAMPSHIRE:
Granite State RLS:
Fran Blakeney, 603-225-2103, GraniteStateRLS@aol.com
Night Walkers of Kendal:
Madith Hamilton, 603-643-2135

NEW MEXICO:
Albuquerque:
Don Tryk, 505-856-6690, dtryk@nmol.com
John Isaminger, 505-293-6723

NEW YORK:
Central New York:
Vincent Lucid, 315-668-8620, DrSpeedbump@email.msn.com
Manhattan:
Marilyn Sachs, 212-684-0565, marilynosp@aol.com
Long Island:
Carol & Bob Germann, 516-735-2295, RLSPLMDLI@aol.com

NORTH CAROLINA:
Greater Western North Carolina:
Doris Walston, 828-668-7180, dww@icu2.net
Raleigh:
Amelia Lewellen, 919-847-7506, rlewellen@mindspring.com

OHIO:
Southwestern:
Jan Schneider, 937-429-0620

OREGON:
Portland:
Cynthia Edwards, 503-297-1932
Salem Hospital:
Delores Johnson, 503-370-5170

PENNSYLVANIA:
Greater Philadelphia:
Edwin & Katheryn Overman, 610-688-5540
Lancaster:
Sally Blair, 717-397-2618

SOUTH CAROLINA:
Midlands:
Joan Waln, 803-356-3444

Texas:
Greater Houston:
Carolyn Achee, 281-361-7366

Helen Simons, 713-468-4192, Hmsimons@aol.com

Vermont:
Southern Vermont:
Eleanor Powers, 802-824-5093

Virginia:
Lynchburg Area:
Pollyanna B. Middleton, 804-384-3216, ARTANdPB@aol.com

Patty Arthur, 804-384-9013, Pararthur@aol.com

Central Virginia:
Pamela Hamilton-Stubbs, MD, 804-354-1163, phstubbsd@hsc.vcu.edu

Washington:
Seattle & Vicinity:
Juanita W. Terrell, 425-746-6925

Susan Bean, 425-885-2604, suzybean@msn.com

Becky Christie, 206-525-8655, Beckyc@u.washington.edu

Olympia:
Kim Chase, 360-493-7436

Spokane Area:
Gene Siverston, 509-448-8424

Eleanor Jones, 509-326-1816

Tacoma Area:
Marian Cooter, 253-582-1069, rlstacwa@yahoo.com

Central Washington:
Ray Gilbert, 509-662-0156, rmg31118@aol.com

Wisconsin:
Fox Cities:
Maxine Welhouse, 920-733-4579

Madison:
Roger Backes, 608-276-4002, roger.backes@mail.mhcdc.org

Jim Albertson, 608-251-6347

CANADA:
Sleep/Wake Canada:
800-387-9253 (calls in Canada)

416-483-9654 (calls from outside Canada)

START AN RLS SUPPORT GROUP

So, you've looked around, you called the national foundation, you checked the list above, you hit the RLS Web site and you still can't find a group anywhere near you. The next step is for you to start an RLS support group yourself.

It isn't hard. First, get in touch with the folks at the RLS Foundation. They have a director of outreach who will help you every step of the way.

Her name is Cindy Stier. Her email address: Stier@rls.org. Or you can send her a snail mail letter at:

> Cindy Stier
> Director of Outreach
> RLS Foundation
> 819 2nd Street SW
> Rochester, MN 55902

She will tell you that leaders not only help those individuals who come to the support group, but during the process the leaders also gain new insights into their own RLS.

The RLS Foundation has some goals they will ask you to strive for:

4 **Increasing universal awareness of RLS.**

4 **Developing effective treatments and ultimately finding a cure for RLS.**

Support groups play an important part in these goals by facilitating discussions about RLS and communicating with family and friends about the disorder.

Each leader of a local RLS support group is asked by the foundation to do these five things:

1. **Be a member in good standing of the Restless Legs Syndrome foundation. Membership fee is $25 a year.**

2. **Complete a volunteer application.**

3. **Participate in a telephone interview with the director of outreach.**

Talk to Cindy Stier about a support group.

4. Contact two established support group leaders.

5. Complete and sign their Memorandum of Understanding.

They have a leadership packet they will send you about becoming a support group leader. If you're interested in doing this in your area, drop the lady an email or a letter.

Until that packet comes, you can still get started. Talk to your doctor and ask if she has any other RLS patients. Explain what you want to do. Chances are that she will help you. A doctor can't give you the names or phone numbers of his RLS patients, but he can give to them or mail to them information about your new group. Put up a color poster about your new group in your doctor's office. Usually the nurses will be glad to help you with this.

If there is a hospital in the area, ask the patient support worker about an RLS group. Tell her what it is and how it works, and ask her if the hospital will provide a room for a meeting. Some will and some won't. Even if they won't loan you the use of a room, most will let you put up notices on their bulletin board for general info about your RLS group.

Try to find out all the doctors in your community who work with RLS patients. Your doctor might be able to help you here. Get a list and then send your RLS first meeting notice to all the doctors in town, announcing the RLS support group. Be sure to list where the meeting will be held, what time, and generally what you hope to do. Explain that this is an organizing meeting, so anyone with ideas about what such a group should do needs to come and get her ideas spelled out.

Let's say the hospital didn't or couldn't loan you a room. Decide to have the meeting in your home. Make it at a convenient time for all. Usually a week

You'll be sent a leadership packet.